PRAYERS

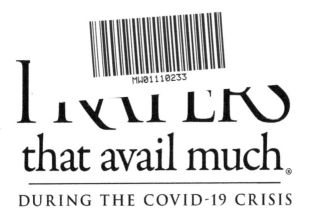

that avail much.®

DURING THE COVID-19 CRISIS

GERMAINE COPELAND

Harrison House

Shippensburg, PA

This is the confidence we have before him: If we ask anything according to his will, he hears us. And if we know that he hears whatever we ask, we know that we have what we have asked of him.

—1 John 5:14-15, CSB

ISBN TP: 978-1-68031-668-1

ISBN eBook: 978-1-68031-669-8

Published by Harrison House
P.O. Box 310
Shippensburg, PA 17257-0310

CONTENTS

A Letter from Germaine to Fellow Believers

Everything has been brought to a halt in our fast-paced world, and it seems as if the earth itself is standing still. Overnight our lives changed as an unseen virus attacked America and far beyond our borders.

BUT GOD!

Hope is still alive and well because God has not changed! He is the same yesterday, today, and forever.

Here on earth we are attempting to find a new normal. Church buildings are closed, and pastors are ministering to their congregations online. School buildings are shuttered. Suddenly parents, children, and teachers are struggling to adjust to changes no one ever anticipated. Non-essential businesses are closed; people are losing their jobs, business owners are trying to survive, and we are faced with unexpected changes. Shoppers walk through stores with empty shelves, and life is presenting us with new opportunities and dilemmas.

We are in a spiritual warfare that I've never experienced before! The atmosphere is filled with a spirit of fear that is spreading across America and around the world. Darkness appears to be settling down over our nation, and I recognize the real enemy of the people: FEAR. Yet, our God has not given us a spirit of fear, but a spirit of power and love and a sound mind.[1] We must submit to Him who is Love and resist fear!

---

1   2 Timothy 1:7

There are two Intercessors who are praying for us—Jesus and the Holy Spirit—and they cannot fail!

Let us arise, devote ourselves to prayer, reinforce our faith, and rejoice in hope of the glory of God. I pray that our love may abound still more and more in knowledge and all discernment, that we may approve the things that are excellent, that we may be sincere and without offense till the day of Christ, being filled with the fruits of righteousness which are by Jesus Christ, to the glory and praise of God.[2]

It's true that our faith has been shaken on many levels, but we are children of God called by His name. He has promised that if, "My people who are called by My name will humble themselves, and pray and seek My face, and turn from their wicked ways,

2   Philippians 1:9-11

then I will hear from heaven, and will forgive their sin and heal their land."[3]

Purpose to believe God! And, therefore, be truly glad! There is wonderful joy ahead, even though you must endure many trials for a little while. These trials will show that your faith is genuine. It is being tested as fire tests and purifies gold—though your faith is far more precious than mere gold. So, when your faith remains strong through many trials, it will bring you much praise and glory and honor on the day when Jesus Christ is revealed to the whole world.[4]

This is our "BUT GOD" moment! The Lord has need of His Church, and we are here for such a time as this. Come with me, and together we will speak scriptural

---

3   2 Chronicles 7:14

4   1 Peter 1:6-8 NLT

prayers into the atmosphere that will stop and still the enemy.

Pray for your family and friends. Share these prayers, write notes, make phone calls. Perfect love casts out fear.

God's Word is forever settled in heaven. And now is the time to forever settle His Word on earth.

Sincerely in His Love,
Germaine

A Declaration of Safety and Security

Be not afraid! Declare, make known, and affirm aloud the Word of the Lord as many times a day as you need to ward off worry! *"I am Your only God, the living God. Wasn't I the one who broke the strongholds over you and raised you up out of bondage? Open your mouth with a mighty decree; I will fulfill it now, you'll see. The words that you speak, so shall it be!"* (Ps. 81:10b TPT)

Below is Psalm 91 personalized from the New Living Translation ready for you to declare your safety and security:

I live in the shelter of the Most High, and I will find rest in the shadow of the

Almighty. This I declare about the LORD: He alone is my refuge, my place of safety. He is my God, and I trust Him.

For He will rescue me from every trap and protect me from deadly disease. He will cover me with His feathers. He will shelter me with His wings. His faithful promises are my armor and protection. I will not be afraid of the terrors of the night, nor the arrow that flies in the day. I do not dread the disease that stalks in darkness, nor the disaster that strikes at midday. Though a thousand fall at my side, though ten thousand are dying around me, these evils will not touch my family or me.

I open my eyes and see how the wicked are punished. If I make the LORD my refuge, if I make the Most High my shelter, no evil will conquer me; no plague will come near my home. For He will order His angels to protect me wherever I go. They will hold me up with their hands so I won't even hurt my foot on a stone. I will trample upon lions and cobras; I will crush fierce lions and serpents under my feet!

The LORD says, "I will rescue those who love Me. I will protect those who trust in My name. When they call on Me, I will answer; I will be with them in trouble. I will rescue and honor them. I will reward them with a long life and give them My salvation."

1

Safety in the Family of God

Father, it is written in Your Word that if I confess with my mouth that Jesus is Lord and believe in my heart that You have raised Him from the dead, I will be saved.

Therefore, Father, I confess that Jesus is my Lord. I make Him Lord of my life right now. I believe in my heart that You raised Jesus from the dead. I renounce my past life with Satan and close the door to any of his devices.

Thank You, Father, for forgiving me of all my sin. Jesus, I declare You as my Savior and Lord! I am a new creation. The past is finished and gone, everything has become fresh and new. The old life is gone; a new life has begun in Jesus' name, amen. Thank You for all You have done for me.

Father, thank You that I have passed from death to life and shall ever be with You, and as a member of the family of God, I enjoy safety and protection in this life here on earth.

SCRIPTURE REFERENCES

John 3:16 • John 14:6 • John 6:37 • Romans 10:9-10 • John 10:10 • Romans 10:13 • Romans 3:23 • Ephesians 2:1-10 • 2 Corinthians 5:19 • 2 Corinthians 5:17 TPT, PHI, NLT • John 16:8-9 • John 1:12 • Romans 5:8 • 1 Corinthians 5:21

2

Healing from Coronavirus

Prayer for the Sick

Father, we pray for those who have been affected by this virus and ask You to surround them with Your presence. You are Jehovah Rapha, who takes sickness out of the midst of them. For those who are struggling to breathe, we ask You to breathe life into their lungs and clear their respiratory systems. Nothing is too hard for You, and nothing is impossible to those who believe. We offer this prayer of faith that will heal the sick. Lord, You will raise them up, and if they have committed sins they will be forgiven, in the name of Jesus. We look to You, the Author and Finisher of our faith.

Prayer for Yourself

Thank You, Father, for sending Your Word to heal me. Jesus, You are the Word who became flesh and lived among us. You bore my griefs (pains) and carried my sorrows (sickness). You were pierced for my transgressions; You were crushed for my iniquities; upon You was the chastisement that brought me peace, and with Your wounds I am healed.

I will fill my thoughts with Your words until they penetrate deep into my spirit. Then, as I unwrap Your words, they will impart true life and radiant health into the very core of my being.

Because Your Spirit who raised Jesus from the dead dwells in me, He who raised Christ from the dead will also give life to my mortal body through Your Spirit who dwells in me.

Scripture References

Exodus 23:25 • Jeremiah 32:17 • Mark 9:23 • James 5:13-20 • Hebrews 12:2 • Proverbs 4:21-22 TPT • 1 Corinthians 6:19-20 • Psalm 103:3-5 • Psalm 107:20 • Romans 8:11 NKJV • John 1:14 • Isaiah 53:4-5 ESV

3

Victory over Fear

Father, when the media gives fear-filled reports about the coronavirus and I feel afraid, I will intentionally choose to put my confidence in You and trust Your promises. You have not given me a spirit of fear but of power and love and self-control.

I have not received a spirit of slavery leading to fear again, but I have received a spirit of adoption as Your child, by which I cry out, "Abba! Father!" I refuse to yield to fear, for You are always near. I set my gaze upon You—the faithful God.

Thank You for infusing me with Your strength and helping me in this fearful situation. You are holding me firmly with Your victorious right hand, and I humbly bow before you, Lord God Almighty.

SCRIPTURE REFERENCES

2 Timothy 1:7 NLT • Romans 8:14-16 CEV
• Isaiah 41:10-12 TPT

4

Letting Go of
Worry and Anxiety

Father, we who are called by Your name humble ourselves under Your mighty hand. Thank You for delivering us from the power of darkness and translating us into the Kingdom of Your dear Son. As your children, we choose to live free from worry in the name of Jesus for the law of the Spirit of life in Christ Jesus has made us free from the law of sin and death. Once we were dead in our trespasses and sins...and lived according to the ruler of the power of the air. But God, who is rich in mercy... made us alive with Christ. By grace we are saved, and You have raised us up with Him and seated us with Him in the heavens in Christ Jesus.

We cry out to You in our distress even as the storm is raging. You are the delivering God, and from Your temple-throne You have heard our troubled cry. We obey Your command and refuse to worry over this worldwide pandemic.

We're here to tell You every detail of our needs in earnest and thankful prayer, and the peace of God, which transcends human understanding, will keep constant guard over our hearts and minds as we rest in Christ Jesus. We believe in goodness and value Your approval. We choose to fix our minds on the things which are holy and right and pure and beautiful and good.

Father-God, we surrender our anxieties. We are silent and choose to stop our striving. You are exalted throughout the whole earth.

Scripture References

1 Peter 5:6 • Colossians 1:13 • Ephesians 2:1-8
CSB • Psalm 18:5-7 TPT • Philippians 4:6-7 PHI
• Psalm 46:10-11

5

Agents of Prayer in
a Time of Crisis

Father, in the name of Jesus, we thank You for calling us to be agents of prayer. We purpose to enter into agreement with the two Intercessors who cannot fail—Jesus and the Holy Spirit. We turn all our worries about coronavirus into prayer.

Jesus, we will never stop trusting You. During this dire trial and tribulation, we commit to pray without ceasing, depending on the Holy Spirit's help.

We choose not to be anxious about anything, but in everything by prayer and supplication with thanksgiving we will let our requests be made known to You. We choose to tell You every detail of the situation then the peace of God will transcend our human understanding. In the name of Jesus, amen.

SCRIPTURE REFERENCES

1 Thessalonians 5:16-18 • Philippians 4:6-7

6

Aligning My Thoughts with God's Word

Father, we are in the world, but we are not of the world. Rather than worry about coronavirus, we choose to believe the report of the Lord. Thank You for the Holy Spirit who guides us into all truth as we bring every thought into proper alignment with the Word of God.

When we hear reports of death and destruction, we are alert to our thoughts, attitudes, and feelings. We are Your children called by Your name, and we purpose to think on things of good report by demolishing every deceptive fantasy that opposes

God. We break through every arrogant attitude raised up in defiance of the true knowledge of God.

Today's reality is not our finality!

You are the Alpha and the Omega—the beginning and the end—the One who is, who always was, and who is still to come! You are the Almighty One!

SCRIPTURE REFERENCES

John 17:11,14 • Isaiah 53:1 • John 16:13 • 2 Corinthians10:4-5 TPT • Psalm 91 • Philippians 4:8 • Revelation 22:13

7

Fight to the Finish

Father, we are here in a fight to the finish! You are strong, and You want us strong. So we take everything You have set out for us, well-made weapons of the best materials. We put them to use so we will be able to stand up to everything the devil is throwing our way. We acknowledge this is no afternoon athletic contest that we'll walk away from and forget about in a couple of hours. This is for keeps, a life-or-death fight to the finish against the devil and all his angels. We are prepared! We're up against far more than we can handle on our own. We take all the help we can get, every weapon You have issued, so that when it's all over but the shouting we'll still be on our feet.

Coronavirus, Marxism, socialism, communism, progressivism, propaganda, media-hype and the occult are no match for truth, righteousness, peace, faith and salvation, which are more than words. We choose to apply them throughout each day. God's Word is an indispensable weapon, and prayer is essential in this ongoing warfare.

With the help of the Holy Spirit, we are here to pray hard and long for our brothers and sisters. Our eyes are open, and we are here to keep each other's spirits up so that no one falls behind or drops out. In the name of Jesus! Amen

SCRIPTURE REFERENCES

Ephesians 6:10-18, MSG

8

Put on Your Armor

Our Father, we are living in a time of great distress and anxiety, and we pray this prayer to remind ourselves of the armor You have provided for us. Therefore, we take unto ourselves the whole armor of God, that we may be able to withstand in the evil day, and having done all, to stand. We stand victorious with the force of Your explosive power flowing in and through us.

Individually, we declare that: My waist is girded with the belt of truth, which contains all the weapons of my warfare. Your weapons are not carnal, but mighty through God to the pulling down of strongholds. I have on the breastplate of righteousness, which is faith and love. My feet are shod with the preparation of the gospel of peace. In Christ Jesus, I have peace and pursue peace with all men. I am a minister of reconciliation, proclaiming the good news of the gospel. I take the shield of faith, where with I am able to quench all the fiery darts of the wicked; the helmet of salvation holding the thoughts, feelings and purposes of Your heart; and the sword of the Spirit, which is the Word of God.

Greater is He that is in me than he that is in the world. I will pray at all times and on every occasion in the name of Jesus!

SCRIPTURE REFERENCES

Ephesians 6:10-18, NKJV, TPT

9

Choose to Rejoice

Father, this is the day You have made. I choose life, and I choose to rejoice and be glad in it! I rejoice in You always—especially during this time of a worldwide pandemic! I choose to delight myself in You, Lord. Happy am I because You are my Lord!

Father, thank You for loving me and rejoicing over me with joy. Hallelujah! I am redeemed, and anxiety is far from me because I fear not! I come with singing and gladness—sorrow and sighing flee away. The spirit of rejoicing, joy, and laughter are my heritage. Where the Spirit of the Lord is, there is liberty—freedom and emancipation from bondage, and I walk in that liberty!

I have the victory in the name of Jesus. Coronavirus, media mind control, and all other devices of the enemy are under my feet. Jesus, You are the Head of the Church. You are my Lord, and I submit to You and will not be moved by adverse circumstances. I dwell in the Kingdom of God, and I have peace and joy in the Holy Spirit in the name of Jesus!

SCRIPTURE REFERENCES

Psalm 118:24 • Deuteronomy 30:19
• Philippians 4:4 • Psalm 100:2 • Isaiah 55:11
• 2 Corinthians 3:17 • Ephesians 1:19-23

10

Ask for God's Wisdom

My Lord and God, You are worthy to receive glory and honor and power, for You created all things. Here in this storm that has come up, the winds of words are raging. Doubt and unbelief are hovering waiting for our response. We choose to count it all joy for we know that the testing of our faith produces steadfastness. This is an opportunity to let steadfastness have its full effect that we may be perfect and complete, lacking in nothing. We resist the temptation to doubt, and with purpose of mind, we ask You for wisdom.

No longer driven and tossed by the wind, we shall remain stable in all our ways during these days of the storm. Father, Your pleasant path leads me to pleasant places. I'm overwhelmed by the privileges that come with following You, for You have given me the best. The way You counsel and correct us makes us praise You more, and Your whispers in the night give us wisdom, showing us what to do next. Thank You for giving us wisdom that is from above in the name of Jesus.

SCRIPTURE REFERENCES

James 1:1-8 • Psalm 16:6-8 TPT

11

Praying for Those
on the Frontlines

Our Father, we thank You for our United States Vice President who asks us to pray for all who are on the frontlines in this time of crisis—the healthcare professionals, the grocery store workers, the police and firefighters, the truck drivers and many more who are working in this environment and then returning home to their families.

We pray for those who are fearful and ask You to protect and defend them. Rescue them and their families from every hidden trap of the enemy and protect them from this deadly curse. We ask You to wrap

Your massive arms around them and protect them from coronavirus in the name of Jesus. Thank You, God, for everyone who is on the frontlines. We choose to make mention of them in our prayers, remembering without ceasing their work of faith and labor of love. Amen.

SCRIPTURE REFERENCES

Psalm 91 TPT • 1 Thessalonians 1:2-3

12

Praying for Our President and Other Leaders

Father, in Jesus' name, we give thanks for the United States and its government. As Your Word exhorts us in 1 Timothy 2:2, we give thanks for all men, for kings, and those in authority that we may lead a quiet and peaceable life.

In the name of Jesus, we come with a prayer of intercession for the President of these United States. We thank You for the person You have appointed for such a time as this. We ask You to give Your servant a discerning heart to govern Your people and to distinguish between right and wrong. We pray that our President will fear the Lord, which is the beginning of wisdom. Wise choices will watch over him and understanding will keep him safe. Wisdom will save him from evil people, from those whose words are twisted.

Father, we pray for godly statesmen/stateswomen who are honorable and of good character. Give our government leaders discernment and keep them from being tricked with foolish talk. May they walk as children of the light exposing greed and corruption. Deliver our nation from evil and from those who oppose Your plan for our nation. Righteousness will guard him whose way is blameless, but wickedness overthrows the sinner.

Give our leaders the courage to submit to You and resist being drawn into doing those worthless things that are done in the dark. *"There is nothing covered that will not be revealed and hidden that will not be known"* (Luke 12:2). Reveal Your will and help them to act with good sense. These are desperate times, and we pray that those You appointed will be strong in You and the power of Your might. Thank You for hearing our prayer!

Jesus is Lord over the United States! Amen.

SCRIPTURE REFERENCES

1 Timothy 2:1-3 • Proverbs 2 • Ephesians 5:6-13
CEV • Proverbs 13:6

13

How to Handle the Day
of Trouble and Calamity

Father, I acknowledge You as my Refuge and High Tower. You are a refuge and a stronghold in these times of trouble, deadly disease, high cost, destitution, and desperation.

In the day of trouble, You will hide me in Your shelter; in the secret place of Your tent will You hide me; You will set me high upon a rock. And now shall my head be lifted up above my enemies round about me; in Your tent I will offer sacrifices and shouting of joy; I will sing, yes, I will sing praises to You.

On the authority of Your Word, I declare that I have been made the righteousness of God in Christ Jesus. When I cry for help, You hear me and deliver me out of all my distress and troubles. Lord, many are the evils that confront me, but You deliver me out of them all.

Thank You for being merciful and gracious to me, for my soul takes refuge and finds shelter and confidence in You; yes, in the shadow of Your wings I take refuge and am confident until calamities and destructive storms are past. You perform on my behalf and reward me. You bring to pass Your purposes for me, and surely You complete them!

God, You're such a safe and powerful place to find refuge! You're a proven help in time of trouble—*more than enough* and always available whenever I need You. So

I will never fear even if every structure of support were to crumble away. I will not fear even when the earth quakes and shakes, moving mountains and casting them into the sea. For the raging roar of stormy winds and crashing waves cannot erode our faith in You.

Lord, like Paul I pleaded with You to relive me of this trouble. I choose to believe Your grace is always more than enough for me and Your power finds its full expression through my weakness. So I celebrate my weaknesses, for when I'm weak I sense more deeply the mighty power of Christ living in me. So I'm not defeated by my weakness, but delighted! For when I feel my weakness and endure mistreatment—when I'm surrounded with troubles on every side and face persecution because of my love for

Christ—I am made yet stronger. For my weakness becomes a portal to Your power.

Lord, You have given me Your peace. By Your grace, I will not let my heart be troubled, neither will I let it be afraid. With the help of the Holy Spirit, I will stop allowing myself to be agitated and disturbed. I refuse to permit myself to be fearful, intimidated, cowardly, and unsettled.

By faith, I respond to these troubles and calamities: I am full of joy now! I exult and triumph in my troubles and rejoice in my sufferings, knowing that pressure and affliction and hardship produce patient and unswerving endurance. And endurance (fortitude) develops maturity of character (approved faith and tried integrity). And character of this sort produces the habit of joyful and confident hope of eternal salvation. Such hope never disappoints or deludes or shames me, for Your love has been poured out in my heart through the Holy Spirit who has been given to me. In Jesus' name, amen.

Scripture References

Psalm 9:9 AMPC • Psalm 57:1-2 AMPC • Psalm 27:5-7 AMPC • Psalm 46:1 TPT • 2 Corinthians 5:21 • 2 Corinthians 12:8-10 TPT • John 14:27 AMPC • Psalm 34:17-20 AMPC • Romans 5:3-5 AMPC

14

God's Help with Finances

Dear Father, I am Your child, and I need Your help in this financial crisis. Whenever I am afraid, I choose to trust You. I feel anxious and out of control. I'm out of work and do not know how I will continue to feed my family and pay the bills. I choose to submit to You. I bind my mind, my will, and my emotions to the will of God. I bind my mind to the truth and to the blood of Jesus. I loose obsessive thinking, anxiety, and fear from my mind. I choose to turn my anxieties into prayer and make my requests known to You.

With the help of the Holy Spirit, I choose not to worry about what my family and I will eat, drink, or what we shall wear, for You know that we need all these things. My family and I seek first the kingdom of God and His righteousness and all these things shall be added to us.

Our Father, Jehovah-Jireh, You are the One who sees our needs and provides for them, and we honor Your name. May the glory of Your name be the center on which our lives turn. Manifest Your kingdom realm and cause Your every purpose to be fulfilled on earth just as it is fulfilled in heaven. We acknowledge You as our Provider of all we need each day.

Forgive us the wrongs we have done as we ourselves release forgiveness to those who have wronged us. Rescue us every time we face tribulations and set us free from evil. For You are the King who rules with power and glory forever.

I am convinced that You, my God, will fully satisfy every need I have, for I have seen the abundant riches of glory *revealed to me* through the Anointed One, Jesus Christ! And God our Father will receive all the glory and the honor throughout the eternity of eternities! Amen!

SCRIPTURE REFERENCES

Psalm 56:3 • Matthew 16:19 • Philippians 4:6 • Matthew 6:9-13 TPT • Philippians 4:19-20 TPT

15

Sweet Sleep

Father, thank You for peaceful sleep and for Your angels that encamp around us who fear You. You deliver us from every sort of harm in this time of crisis to keep us safe. The angels excel in strength, do Your word, and heed the voice of Your Word.

You give Your angels charge over me, to keep me in all my ways.

I bring every thought, every imagination, and every dream into the captivity and obedience of Jesus Christ. Father, I thank You that, even as I sleep, my heart counsels me and reveals to me Your purpose and plan. Thank You for sweet sleep, for You promised Your beloved sweet sleep. Therefore, my heart is glad and my spirit rejoices. My body and soul rest and confidently dwell in safety. In Jesus' name, amen.

SCRIPTURE REFERENCES

Proverbs 3:24 • Psalm 91:11 • Psalm 34:7 • 2 Corinthians 10:5 • Psalm 103:20

16

Pleading the Blood of Jesus

Father, I plead the blood of Jesus upon my life—within me, around me, and between me and all evil and the author of evil. I plead the blood of Jesus on all property that belongs to me and on all over which You have made me a steward.

I plead the blood of Jesus on the portals of my mind, my body (the temple of the Holy Spirit), my emotions, and my will. I believe that I am protected by the blood of the Lamb, which gives me access to the Holy of Holies.

I plead the blood over my spouse, my children, my grandchildren and their children, and on all my family that You have given me in this life.

Lord, You have said that the life of the flesh is in the blood. Thank You for this blood that has cleansed me from sin and sealed the New Covenant of which I am a partaker. In Jesus' name, amen.

SCRIPTURE REFERENCES

Exodus 12:7,13 • Leviticus 17:11
• 1 Corinthians 6:19 • 1 John 1:7 • Hebrews 9:6-14
• Hebrews 13:20 AMPC

17

Renewing Your Mind

Father, thank You that I shall prosper and be in health, even as my soul prospers. I have the mind of Christ, the Messiah, and do hold the thoughts, feelings, and purposes of His heart. I trust in You, Lord, with all my heart; I lean not unto my own understanding, but in all of my ways I acknowledge You. You shall direct my paths.

Today I submit myself to Your Word, which exposes and sifts and analyzes and judges the very thoughts and purposes of my heart. For the weapons of my warfare are not carnal, but mighty through You to the pulling down of strongholds—intimidation, fears, doubts, unbelief, and failure. I refute arguments and theories and reasonings and every proud and lofty thing that sets itself up against the true knowledge of God. I lead every thought and purpose away captive into the obedience of Christ, the Messiah, the Anointed One.

Today I shall be transformed by the renewing of my mind, that I may prove what is that good and acceptable and perfect will of God. Your Word, Lord, shall not depart out of my mouth; but I shall meditate on it day and night, that I may observe to do according to all that is written therein—for then I shall make my way prosperous, then I shall have good success.

My thoughts are the thoughts of the diligent, which lead to abundance. Therefore, I am not anxious about anything, but in everything, by prayer and petition, with thanksgiving, I present my requests to God.

And the peace of God, which transcends all understanding, will guard my heart and my mind in Christ Jesus.

Today I fix my mind on whatever is *true*, whatever is *worthy of reverence* and is *honorable* and *seemly*, whatever is *just*, whatever is *pure*, whatever is *lovely* and *lovable*, whatever is *kind* and *winsome* and *gracious*. If there is any *virtue* and *excellence*, if there is anything *worthy of praise*, I will think on and weigh and take account of these things.

Today I roll my works upon You, Lord. I commit and trust them wholly to You. You will cause my thoughts to become agreeable to Your will, and so shall my plans be established and succeed. In Jesus' name I pray, amen.

SCRIPTURE REFERENCES

3 John 2 • Romans 12:2 • 1 Corinthians 2:16
AMPC • Joshua 1:8 • Proverbs 3:5-6 • Proverbs
21:5 ESV • Hebrews 4:12 AMPC • Philippians
4:6-8 NIV • 2 Corinthians 10:4-5 AMPC
• Proverbs 16:3 AMPC

18

Praying for the Health and Safety of Loved Ones

Father, thank You that You watch over Your Word to perform it. Thank You that as my family dwells in the secret place of the Most High, they remain stable and fixed under the shadow of the Almighty, whose power no foe can withstand.

You are my family's Refuge and Fortress. No evil shall befall my spouse or my children. No accident shall overtake them—nor any plague or calamity come near our home. You give Your angels special charge over us to accompany and defend and preserve us in all our ways. They are encamped around about us.

Father, You are my family's Confidence, firm and strong. You keep their feet from hidden danger. *Jesus is their Safety!*

I surround my spouse and my children with faith in You and the power of Your Word. You will rescue them from every hidden trap of the enemy and protect them from false accusations and any deadly curse. Your massive arms are wrapped around them, protecting them wherever they may be. Wherever they go, Your hand will guide them; Your strength will empower them. It is impossible for them to disappear from You or to ask the darkness to hide them, for Your presence is everywhere, bringing light into their night.

Lord, Your name is so great and powerful! People everywhere see Your splendor. Your glorious majesty streams from the heavens, filling the earth with the fame of Your name! You have built a stronghold by the songs of babies. Strength rises up with the chorus of singing children. This kind of praise has the power to shut Satan's mouth. Child-like worship will silence the madness of those who oppose You. We are in awe of Your majesty! We are in awe of such great power and might!

The enemy is turned back from my family in the name of Jesus! They increase in wisdom and in favor with God and man. In Jesus' name, amen.

SCRIPTURE REFERENCES

Ezekiel 22:30 • Proverbs 4:1-15 TPT • Genesis 18:19 • Psalm 119:11 TPT • Psalm 127:4-5 TPT • 3 John 4 • Psalm 91 TPT, AMPC • Psalm 139:10-11 TPT • Psalm 81:1-12 TPT • Psalm 29:2 TPT • Jeremiah 1:12 • Proverbs 3:23-24 AMPC • Psalm 112:7 • Isaiah 26:3 • Psalm 149:5 • Psalm 34:7 • Psalm 3:5 • Proverbs 3:26 AMPC • Psalm 4:8 AMPC • Isaiah 49:25 • Mark 4:35 • Psalm 127:2

19

Hedge of Protection

Father, we lift up _____ to You and pray a hedge of protection around him/her. We thank You, Father, that You are a wall of fire round about _____ and that You set Your angels round about him/her.

We thank You, Father, that _____ dwells in the secret place of the Most High and abides under the shadow of the Almighty. We say of You, Lord, You are his/her refuge and fortress, in You will he/she trust. You cover _____ with Your feathers, and under Your wings shall he/she trust. _____ shall not be afraid of the terror by night or the arrow that flies by day.

Only with his/her eyes will _____ behold and see the reward of the wicked.

Because _____ has made You, Lord, his/her Refuge and Fortress, no evil shall befall him/her—no accident will overtake him/her—neither shall any plague or calamity come near him/her. For You give Your angels charge over _____, to keep him/her in all Your ways.

Father, because You have set Your love upon _____, therefore will You deliver him/her. _____shall call upon You, and You will answer him/her. You will be with him/her in trouble and will satisfy _____with a long life and show him/her Your salvation. Not a hair of his/her head shall perish. Amen.

SCRIPTURE REFERENCES

Ezekiel 22:30 • Psalm 91:4-5 AMPC

• Zechariah 2:5 • Psalm 91:8-11 AMPC

• Psalm 34:7 • Psalm 91:14-16 AMPC

• Psalm 91:1-2 AMPC • Luke 21:18

20

Protection and
Deliverance of a City

Father, in the name of Jesus, we have
received Your power—ability, efficiency,
and might—because the Holy Spirit has
come upon us. We are Your witnesses in
_____ and to the ends, the very
bounds, of the earth.

Father, we confidently and boldly draw
near to Your throne of grace, that we may
receive mercy and find grace to help in time
of need on behalf of the city of _____
_____. Thank You for sending forth Your
commandments to the earth. Your Word

runs very swiftly throughout _____
and continues to grow and spread.

Father, we seek the peace and welfare of
_____, where You have planted us
to live. We pray to You for the welfare of
this city and do our part by getting involved
in it. We pray for every political leader and
representative, so that we would be able to
live tranquil, undisturbed lives, as we worship You, the awe-inspiring God, with pure
hearts. It pleases You that we pray for them,
for You long for everyone to embrace Your
life and return to the full knowledge of
the truth.

Holy Spirit, we ask You to make us good
citizens, for all governments are under
God. Insofar as there is peace and order,
it's God's order. Help us to live responsibly
as citizens, for decent citizens should have
nothing to fear.

Father, we pray for deliverance and salvation for those who are following the course and fashion of this world—who are under the sway of the tendency of this present age—following the prince of the power of the air. Father, forgive them, for they know not what they do.

In Jesus' mighty name we break the power of the devil, the god of this world, who has blinded the minds of those who don't believe and have not received the glorious light of the good news. We pray that the Lord of the harvest send laborers across their paths with the Gospel of Jesus Christ. We pray that the Father of glory, the God of our Lord Jesus Christ, would impart to them the riches of the Spirit of wisdom and the Spirit of revelation to know Him through deepening intimacy. May their hearts be flooded with light until they experience the wealth of God's glorious inheritances.

Thank You, Father, for the guardian angels assigned to this place who war for us in the heavenlies. In the name of Jesus, we stand victorious over the principalities, powers, rulers of the darkness of this world, and spiritual wickedness in high places over _____.

We ask the Holy Spirit to sweep through the gates of our city and convince the people and bring demonstration to them about sin and about righteousness—uprightness of heart and right standing with God.

Father, You said, "For I know the thoughts and plans that I have for you... thoughts and plans for welfare and peace and not for evil, to give you hope in your final outcome" (Jer. 29:11 AMPC). By the

blessing of the influence of the upright and God's favor because of them, the city of
_____ is exalted. Amen.

SCRIPTURE REFERENCE

Acts 1:8 AMPC • Ephesians 1:17-23 TPT
• Hebrews 4:16 AMPC • 2 Corinthians 4:4
AMPC • Psalm 147:15 AMPC • Ephesians 6:12
• Acts 12:24 AMPC • Jeremiah 29:7-8 AMPC
• John 16:8 AMPC • Romans 13:1-7 MSG
• Jeremiah 29:11 AMPC • Matthew 9:37-38
• Proverbs 11:11 AMPC • Ephesians 2:2 AMPC
• 1 Timothy 2:2-4 TPT

21

A Heart for the Lost

Father, during this time of crisis, we come to stand in the gap before You and pray for those who are lost. The lost are always on our hearts—as they are Yours. But in this hour, we are ever aware that the greatest risk is not to be infected by a virus but to be lost and without You eternally. We pray in agreement with Jesus who is able to save to the uttermost those who come to You through Him because He always lives to make intercession for them.

We pray for those who are perishing, for their minds are blinded by the god of this age, leaving them in unbelief. Open their blind eyes that keep them from seeing the dayspring light of the wonderful news of the glory of Jesus Christ. Father, let Your brilliant light shine out of darkness and cascade Your light into them that they might see the knowledge of grace and truth.

We are here to take our stand against the unseen spirits of darkness that have held them in bondage. We pray for their deliverance from the power of darkness and ask You to convey them into the kingdom of the Son of Your love, in whom we have redemption through His blood, the forgiveness of sins.

Father, we know that Satan would prevent these people from hearing truth, if possible. We are human, but we don't wage war with human plans and methods. We use God's mighty weapons to knock down the devil's strongholds. With these weapons we break down every proud argument that keeps people from confessing Jesus as Lord and believing in their hearts that You raised Him from the dead. We pray the people will be saved and come to the knowledge of the truth.

When the Light shines out of darkness, and they hear the good news of the gospel, they will call upon the name of the Lord and be saved. Thank You for loving us even when we were Your enemies. You gave Your Son, Your one and only Son, so that no one need be destroyed; by believing in Him, anyone can have a whole and lasting life.

Jesus, You are not late with Your promise to return. The delay reveals Your loving patience toward those who do not yet know You because You do not want any to perish but all to come to repentance.

Lord Jesus, when we look at the nations, we realize that the harvest of souls is huge and ripe! We ask the Owner of the harvest to thrust out many more reapers to harvest His grain!

We confess that they shall see who have never been told of Jesus. They shall understand who have never heard of Jesus. And they shall come out of the snare of the devil who has held them captive. They shall open their eyes and turn from darkness to light—from the power of Satan to You, God! In Jesus' name, amen.

Scripture References

Hebrews 7:25 NKJV • 2 Corinthians 4:1-6 TPT • 1 Corinthians 10:3-5 NLT • Romans 15:21 AMPC • Matthew 9:38 • 2 Timothy 2:26 AMPC • Colossians 1:13 NKJV • 2 Peter 3:8-10 TPT

22

Prayer for Our Citizens

Our Father-God, we come before You to stand in the gap and build up the hedge on behalf of America during this time of crisis. Our trust is in You, and we believe that if we who are called by Your name will humble ourselves, and pray and seek Your face, and turn from our wicked ways, then You will hear from heaven and will forgive our sin and heal our land.

We pray for the people of this great nation. As we pray, we choose to forgive those who have turned their backs on our God and our history. Lead them by Your Spirit to repentance by Your goodness. It is our prayer that Your Word will run swiftly throughout every city and village of this country. Holy Spirit, we thank You for giving our government officials a spirit of counsel and wisdom so that they may communicate a message of hope for this country. You give the wise answers, and we pray that their words will be a demonstration of Your wisdom operating in them. In the name of Jesus, we pull down the stronghold of deception working to entrap the people. Father, watch over everyone who shows good sense, and frustrate the plans of deceitful liars. We decree and declare that truth shall prevail!

Prepare the hearts of the citizens to hear words that will persuade them that Your will must be done in our nation and then we will fulfill our destiny. We pray that in a time of trouble men's hearts will not fail them, but they will continue in faith. We pray that You will give us, the citizens of heaven and America, the discerning of the signs of the times. Give the people of this nation a spirit of wisdom and revelation in the knowledge of You. May our prayers for this nation release rivers of living water for the healing of America in the name of Jesus. Amen.

SCRIPTURE REFERENCES

Ephesians 1:17-19 • 2 Chronicles 7:14
• 2 Timothy 2:1 • Romans 2:4

23

Prayer for Grieving Families

Our Father, in the name of Jesus, we are here to pray for those who are grieving the loss of a loved one. Jehovah-Adonai, You are the completely self-existing One who is always present. We bless You, Father of mercies and God of all comfort, who comforts my friends in this time of grief.

They are certain about the truth concerning those who have passed away, so that they won't be overwhelmed with grief like many others who have no hope. We believe that Jesus died and rose again; we also believe that God will bring with Jesus those who died while believing in Him. This is the word of the Lord: we who are alive in

Him and remain on earth when the Lord appears will by no means have an advantage over those who have already died, for both will rise together.

Thank You for sending the Holy Spirit to comfort, counsel, help, intercede, defend, strengthen, and stand by my friends as only He can in their time of grief and sorrow in the name of Jesus.

SCRIPTURE REFERENCES

2 Corinthians 1:3-5 • 1 Thessalonians 4:13-18 TPT • John 14:26 AMPC

24

Redeeming the Time
while Sheltered-in-Place

Abba-Father, we are Your people who are sheltered-in-place. Now that our doors are shut, we will wait until this indignation is past. With the help of the Holy Spirit, we will look carefully at how we are to walk with one another. We will encourage others with phone calls and handwritten notes.

Holy Spirit, we purpose to live worthily and accurately—taking care of our bodies, which are the temples of the Holy Spirit. We go for walks where we stand in awe, startled and stunned by signs and wonders. Sunrise brilliance and sunset beauty both take turns singing their songs of joy to You. In the quietness of the day, we will praise You for Your magnificent greatness, praise You with musical instruments and song!

As I organize my home and my surroundings, I let go of worry about missing out, and my everyday concerns will be met. As I work from home, I thank You for giving me a spirit of self-discipline that I might work expediently and take reasonable breaks.

In my quite times, I invite Your searching gaze into my heart. Examine me through and through; find out everything that may be hidden within me. Put me to the test and sift through all my anxious cares. See if there is any path of pain I'm walking on and lead me back to Your glorious, everlasting ways—the path that brings me back to You in the name of Jesus.

SCRIPTURE REFERENCES

Isaiah 26:20 NKJV • Psalm 65:8 TPT
• Psalm 150 • Psalm 139:23-24 TPT

25

Be the Church

Father, our lives have been turned upside down during this time of crisis, and we are looking to You for support and guidance. We honor our pastors and thank You that they care for us and have been examples that we can follow as they follow Jesus.

As Christians, though we are many, we've all been mingled into one body in Christ. This means that we are all vitally joined to one another—each contributing to the others.

With the help of the Holy Spirit, we choose to seize this moment to help people, pray for people, and shine forth Your glory without fear! Help us provide practical help to the lonely and those who are anxious and hurting—whether it be running errands or reaching out with phone calls, text messages, or handwritten notes. We are your representatives here on earth, and by the grace imparted to us, we will walk in love as children of light and in the wisdom of God. We are here to buy up every opportunity for Your glory and honor.

We desire to be the Church and strengthen and build up others in all ways—spiritually, socially, and materially. Alert us, Holy Spirit, to opportunities where we can encourage, admonish, exhort, and edify others. We purpose to reach out to parents, students who are learning at home, single people who live alone, grandparents, and widows and widowers. O Lord, there are so many needs!

Here I am, Lord, use me—I desire to be the Church.

I purpose to do for others what I desire others would do for me. In Your Church, Lord, be glorified, in the name of Jesus and by the power of the Holy Spirit.

SCRIPTURE REFERENCES

Romans 12:3-5 TPT • Romans 15:2 AMPC
• Hebrews 10:13 • Luke 6:31

26

Standing Strong in the Lord

LORD, You are my light and my salvation—so why should I be afraid? You are my Fortress, protecting me from danger!

When enemies and foes attack us, they will stumble and fall. United in prayer with my brothers and sisters, and clothed in the armor of God, we take our stand against the Luciferian spirit that is attempting to overthrow the plans of our God for America. Today, we proclaim our Lord destroys the plans and spoils the schemes of enemy nations and the forces of darkness.

Jesus arose victorious over death and the grave! What the Lord has planned will

Prayers That Avail Much₂ During the COVID-19 Crisis

stand forever! This coronavirus has come to steal, kill, and destroy, but we choose life, proclaiming Jesus has come that we might have life and have it more abundantly! Some find their strength in their weapons and wisdom, but America's miracle deliverance can never be won by men. Our boast is in the Lord our God, who makes us strong and gives us victory!

Our enemies will not prevail; they will only collapse and perish in defeat while we will rise up, full of courage in the name of Jesus.

Scripture References

Psalm 27:1-2 • Ephesians 6:12 • John 10:10
• Psalm 20:7-8 TPT

104

27

Financial Recovery after Coronavirus and Lockdown

Our Father in heaven, we bless Your holy name. Your kingdom come; Your will be done on earth as it is in heaven. In Jesus' name we call for powerful leaders who will speak truly, live truly, and deal truly; who will walk in integrity in trade and commerce.

We pray they will recognize You in all their deliberations and ask You for wisdom that only You can give. We pray they will make judgments in their gates that are for truth, justice, and peace. May they be a people who lean not unto their own understanding, but in all their ways they will learn to acknowledge You, and You shall direct their paths.

Give them creative ideas as they promote the proper flow and balance of the production of resources, the distribution of resources, and the consumption of resources. We ask You to give us unpresumptuous economic leaders who trust in the living God, who ask for and receive wisdom and understanding.

Father, thank You for appointing and anointing leaders who live under the banner of the Lord's provision. Today, we lift up Wall Street, the bankers, and the economists, praying they will do according to all that You have commanded us. It is our prayer that these leaders will be governed by the law of love, giving tithes and offerings, and they will feed the hungry and give them something to drink; they will welcome strangers, shelter and clothe them, provide help for the sick and infirmed, and minister to those in prison in the name of Jesus.

SCRIPTURE REFERENCES

Matthew 6:9-10 • Ephesians 4:15 • Proverbs 3:5-6 • Zechariah 8:16-18 • Matthew 25:35

28

Repentance for the Body of Christ

Our Father, we are Your people called by Your name. We humble ourselves, pray, and seek Your face. We choose to turn from our wicked ways. We ask You to come and heal our land. Thank You that we have a forgiving Redeemer who is face-to-face with You. Jesus is the atoning sacrifice for our sins, and not only for ours but also for the sins of the whole world.

We confess that we allowed our minds to be diverted by the schemes of the enemy, justified blaming others for our failures, and we have sinned against You with our words spoken contrary to Your will. Forgive us for taking up the offenses of the past sins and blaming our ungodly attitude of unforgiveness on those who have wronged us. We will stand before You at the day of judgment and give an account for our personal deeds.

Forgive us for holding others to a higher standard than we hold ourselves. Forgive us for voting contrary to life and godliness.

We raise up the banner of love and take our stand against the accuser, the father of lies who uses racism and the pain of the past to separate us from unity. Because of our deepest respect and worship of God, we remove everything from our lives that contaminates body and spirit, and we choose to complete the development of holiness within us in the name of Jesus. We are a people whose identity is in Christ, and by the power of the Holy Spirit, we will walk together clothed in the armor of God.

SCRIPTURE REFERENCES

2 Chronicles 7:14 • 1 John 2:1-2

29

Prayer Against Terrorism

Father, we praise You and offer up thanksgiving because Jesus is coming soon. We are here to take our stand against the evil spirits of terrorism, which have come to steal, kill, and destroy. Thank You for the Holy Spirit who rises up within us to super-intercede on our behalf. We are here pleading to You with emotional sighs too deep for words. Father God, You are the searcher of the heart, and You know fully our longings, yet You also understand the desires of the Spirit because the Holy Spirit is passionately pleading before You for us, Your holy ones, in perfect harmony with Your plan and our destiny.

Therefore, we will not fret or have any anxiety about terrorism threatening the lives of unsuspecting and innocent people. We submit to You and resist the temptation to be pulled in different directions or worried about a thing. We are saturated in prayer throughout each day, offering our faith-filled requests before You with overflowing gratitude.

Father, our petition is that terrorism in the heavenlies and on earth be stopped! You have not given us a spirit of fear, but a spirit of love, power, and a sound mind. Therefore, we will not be in fear of those who can kill only the body but not our souls.

Lord, You know where every terrorist cell is located across this nation. Father, I ask You to cut asunder the cords of this wicked net (Ps. 129:4). And bring disarray, confusion, defection, and a holy fear of God into the enemy camp. Sever their communication network, their financial funding, and their tracking systems. Diffuse their power and expose their evil schemes and terrorist activities and bring them to justice, in Jesus' name.

Father, I pray that You would target every terrorist leader, and that like Saul of Tarsus, You would knock them off their "high horses" of pride, delusion, and deception. May the brilliance of Your Glory surround them and bring them to their knees in surrender to You! (Acts 9:1-6). I push back the occult cover of darkness that conceals them. For it is written: "Their webs of evil will not become garments; or will they cover themselves with their works." I declare in Jesus' name that their works will be exposed, and the perpetrators apprehended, for theirs are "works of iniquity, and the act of violence is in their hands" (Isa. 49:6).

Father, we offer this prayer to You in the name of Jesus, amen.[1]

SCRIPTURE REFERENCES

Philippians 4:5-6 TPT • Romans 8:31 • Luke 10:19 AMPC • 2 Timothy 1:7 AMPC • Ephesians 6:10 AMPC • Psalm 91:5-6 AMPC • Ephesians 2:2 AMPC • Isaiah 54:14 AMPC • Ephesians 6:12 AMPC • Proverbs 3:3 AMPC • Matthew 16:19 • Psalm 50:23 • Psalm 56:9 AMPC • Romans 8:26-27 TPT

---

1   Quoted with permission from Intercessors for America, IFApray.org.

30

Protection in Destructive Weather and Natural Disaster

Father, we are ever grateful that not one word of Your good promise has ever failed to come to pass. You are a loving Father who is good and faithful to Your children. You protect us from every sort of evil in Jesus' name.

Earthquakes, famines, hurricanes, tornadoes, droughts, fires, tsunamis, floods, and more are the results of sin and its effects on a planet that is groaning and travailing in pain under the bondage of corruption.

You gave the earth to man and woman, who were to fill it and govern it. Through Adam's disobedience, suffering and death were unleashed upon the human race. In some cases, man's own neglect of our planet has brought harm to planet Earth. Father, the devil is called the god of this world, but we know that Jesus defeated him when He was raised from the dead! Dear Father, You have imparted to us the same mighty power that raised Christ from the dead and seated Him in the place of honor at Your right hand in the heavenly realms.

During the flood in the days of Noah, the planet was shaken to its core—dramatically altered from Your original design. Now these natural disasters and weather patterns bring death and destruction to millions. But we know, Father, that You do not send them. Every gift from You is good, perfect, and wholesome, streaming down from above. You are the Father of lights who shines from the heavens with no hidden shadow or darkness and is never subject to change.

We cannot control the events that transpire in this fallen world. We cannot declare there will be no more natural disasters or destructive weather. Your Word even predicts these events as we draw closer to the return of Jesus. You said "there will be terrible earthquakes—seismic events of epic proportion, horrible epidemics and famines in place after place. This is how the first contractions and birth pains of the new age will begin" (Matt. 24:7-8 TPT).

But, Father, we thank You that we can prevent them from coming to our homes and our property. We can minimize their damage with our prayers and our words.

We can rebuke the wind and the waves and speak "peace be still" to storms just as Jesus did (Mark 4:37-41). We can speak to the elements just as Elijah did (see James 5:17-18). And we can receive Your safety and protection!

Father, thank You for the first responders who lay down their lives for others. Be a shield round about them as they go to rescue those who need help. When floods roar like thunder and lift their pounding waves, we shout to You, our God. You are mightier than the violent raging of the seas, mightier than the breakers on the shore—You, Lord, are mightier than these! You are a present help in time of trouble.

Thank You for the provisions of Psalm 91 (TPT). We pray Your promises of protection over our lives, proclaiming: My family and I sit enthroned under the shadow of

Shaddai. We are hidden in Your strength, God Most High. You are the hope that holds us and the Stronghold that shelters us. You are the only God for us and our great confidence. You rescue us from every hidden trap of the enemy and protect us from false accusation and any deadly curse. Your massive arms are wrapped around us, protecting us. We can run under Your covering of majesty and hide. Your arms of faithfulness are a shield keeping us from harm.

We will never worry about an attack of demonic forces at night, nor will we fear a spirit of darkness coming against us. We don't fear a thing!

Whether by night or by day, demonic danger will not trouble us, nor will the powers of evil launch against us.

Even in a time of disaster, with thousands and thousands being killed, we will remain unscathed and unharmed. We will be a spectator as the wicked perish in judgment, for they will be paid back for what they have done! When we live our lives within Your shadow, Most High, our secret hiding place, we will always be shielded from harm. How then could evil prevail against us or disease infect us? It cannot!

Thank You for sending angels with special orders to protect us wherever we go, defending us from all harm. If we walk into a trap, they'll be there for us and keep us from stumbling. We even walk unharmed among the fiercest powers of darkness, trampling every one of them beneath our feet!

For here is what You have spoken: "Because you have delighted in me as my great lover, I will greatly protect you. I will set you in a high place, safe and secure before my face. I will answer your cry for help every time you pray, and you will find and feel my presence even in your time of pressure and trouble. I will be your glorious hero and give you a feast. You will be satisfied with a full life and with all that I do for you. For you will enjoy the fullness of my salvation!" (Ps. 91:14-16 TPT). In Jesus' name we pray, amen.

Scripture References

2 Kings 5:8 • 1 Kings 8:56 • James 1:17 TPT
• Romans 8:21-22 WEB • Psalm 93:3-4 NLT •
Psalm 115:16 • Psalm 107:20 NKJV • Psalm 8:4-6
•Matthew 24:7 TPT • Genesis 1:26-28
• Mark 4:37-41 • 2 Corinthians 4:4 • James 5:17-18
• Hebrews 2:14 • Psalm 91 TPT • Ephesians 2:6

31

The Best Is Yet to Come

Our Father, You keep all Your promises.
We treasure Your commands and tune our
ears to wisdom and understanding. Then
we will understand what it means to fear
the Lord. Wise choices will watch over
us and understanding will keep us safe.
Even as the winds of coronavirus and other
unknown forces of darkness are raging, we
choose to fear You. Our faith is not in the
virus but in You. Even when there is something to fear—we choose to believe Your
promises to us. Your plans are for our welfare and not for evil, to give us a future and
a hope. You caused us to be born again to
a living hope through the resurrection of
Jesus Christ from the dead.

We know the sufferings of this present time are not worth comparing with the glory that is to be revealed to us. We choose to rejoice in hope, to be patient in tribulation, and constant in prayer for the best is yet to come.

You are the God of hope filling us with all joy and peace in believing, so that by the power of the Holy Spirit we may abound in hope! Our citizenship is in heaven, and from it we await a Savior, the Lord Jesus Christ. And now, Lord, where do I put my hope? My only hope is in You!

The steadfast love of the Lord never ceases. His mercies never come to an end; they are new every morning. Great is Your faithfulness. The best is yet to come!

SCRIPTURE REFERENCES

Psalm 146:1 • Proverbs 2 • Jeremiah 29:11
• 1 Peter 1:3-4 • Romans 12:12 • Romans 8:18
• Philippians 3:20 • Psalm 39:7 NLT
• Lamentations 3:21-23

About Germaine Copeland

Germaine Copeland is the author of the bestselling *Prayers That Avail Much*® book series. Founder and president of Word Ministries, Inc., Germaine has traveled nationally and internationally conducting prayer schools and speaking at churches and conferences. Today, her ministry reaches around the world through her books and teaching videos. Germaine and her husband, Everette, have four children, eleven grandchildren, and a growing number of great-grandchildren and great-great grandchildren.

Mission Statement

Word Ministries, Inc.

To motivate individuals to spiritual growth and emotional wholeness, encouraging them to become more deeply and intimately acquainted with Father God as they pray prayers that avail much.

Contact Word Ministries by writing:

Word Ministries, Inc.

P. O. Box 289

Good Hope, GA 30641

(770) 267-7603

www.prayers.org

Other Bestselling Books in the
Prayers That Avail Much® series

*Prayers That Avail Much® 40th Anniversary
Gift Edition*

*Prayers That Avail Much® Gold-Letter
Gift Edition*

Prayers That Avail Much® Volume 1

A Global Call to Prayer

Prayers That Avail Much® for New Believers

Prayers That Avail Much® for Your Family

*Prayers That Avail Much® for Women –
pocket edition*

*Prayers That Avail Much® for Men –
pocket edition*

Prayers That Avail Much ® for Parents

*Prayers That Avail Much® for Moms –
pocket edition*

Prayers That Avail Much® for Mothers

Prayers That Avail Much® for Grandparents

Prayers That Avail Much® for Young Adults

Prayers That Avail Much® for the College Years

Prayers That Avail Much® for Teens

Prayers That Avail Much® for the Workplace

Prayers That Avail Much® for Leaders

*Prayers That Avail Much®
365-Day Devotional*

Prayers That Avail Much® for America

Prayers That Avail Much® for the Nations

Prayers That Avail Much® for Graduates

The Harrison House Vision

Proclaiming the truth and the power
of the Gospel of Jesus Christ with excellence.
Challenging Christians
to live victoriously,
grow spiritually,
know God intimately.

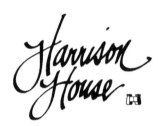

Connect with us on

f Facebook @ HarrisonHousePublishers

and 🄾 Instagram @ HarrisonHousePublishing

so you can stay up to date with news

about our books and our authors.

Visit us at **www.harrisonhouse.com**

for a complete product listing as well as

monthly specials for wholesale distribution.

CPSIA information can be obtained
at www.ICGtesting.com
Printed in the USA
LVHW011645280620
659167LV00013B/667